Diabetes Recipe Cookbook For Beginners

Delicious Recipes for healthy and proper Control of High Blood Sugar level.

Dr. Emmzy

Table of content

Breakfast Options

 Chapter 17
Slow Cooker and Instant Pot Recipes for Convenient Cooking
 Slow cookers and Instant Pots have transformed food preparation, giving ease, adaptability, and tasty results with no effort. In this chapter, we'll explore a range of delectable dishes customised for these practical cooking machines, from rich stews to tender meats and nourishing soups.

Chapter 18
Meal Planning Tips and Strategies for Long-Term Blood Sugar Management

Introduction

Welcome to the "Diabetes Recipe Cookbook for Beginners," a comprehensive resource offering delectable meals suitable for individuals with diabetes, aiming to transform their dietary habits and overall lifestyle.

Managing diabetes can be daunting, but it can be overcome. This book transcends being a mere compilation of recipes; it serves as a guide towards a more robust and contented version of yourself. Whether a someone has recently received a diagnosis or seeks to update their culinary skills, this cookbook serves as a reliable resource in the pursuit of improved well-being.

Within these pages, you will encounter a wealth of delectable recipes meticulously crafted with a focus on novices. Each recipe is meticulously designed to assist individuals in managing their diabetes while maintaining taste and enjoyment, encompassing a range of meals from substantial breakfasts to gratifying dinners and enticing sweets.

However, this book examines not just the content of your meals, but also the manner in which you consume them.

By providing practical advice, dietary recommendations, and meal planning techniques, we want to enable individuals to assume responsibility for their well-being and make informed decisions on a daily basis.

Let us commence this gastronomic expedition collectively. Let's rediscover the joy of cooking and eating, one delicious recipe at a time. Are you ready to embrace a life filled with flavor, vigor, and well-being? Then let's dig in and experience the transforming power of food.

Chapter 1

Understanding Diabetes and Blood Sugar Impact

A. Overview of Diabetes Types.

Diabetes is a chronic condition characterised by high levels of glucose in the blood, either due to inadequate insulin production, resistance to insulin's effects, or both. There are various forms of diabetes, each with its own causes and care strategies:

Type 1 diabetes: This type is an autoimmune disease in which the body's immune system mistakenly assaults and destroys the insulin-producing beta cells in the pancreas. As a result, the body generates little or no insulin, leading to excessive blood sugar levels.

Type 2 Diabetes: In type 2 diabetes, the body becomes resistant to insulin or doesn't create enough insulin to maintain normal blood sugar levels. This form of diabetes is commonly related to lifestyle factors such as obesity, physical inactivity, and a poor diet.

Gestational diabetes: This kind of diabetes occurs during pregnancy and normally resolves after childbirth. However, women who have experienced gestational diabetes are at a higher risk of having type 2 diabetes later in life.

B. Impact of Diet on Blood Sugar

Diet has a significant role in managing diabetes by regulating blood sugar levels. Carbohydrates, in particular, have the most substantial impact on blood glucose, as they are converted into sugar during digestion. Other nutrients, such as protein and fat, also affect blood sugar levels, albeit to a lesser extent.

Carbohydrates: Foods rich in carbohydrates, such as bread, pasta, rice, and sweet snacks, can cause blood sugar levels to rise rapidly. It's vital for patients with diabetes to check their carbohydrate intake and choose sources that have a minimum influence on blood sugar, such as whole grains, fruits, and vegetables.

Protein: Protein-rich foods, such as lean meats, poultry, fish, tofu, and lentils, have a low influence on blood sugar levels and can assist improve satiety and weight management.

Fat: While fats do not directly alter blood sugar levels, they do influence insulin sensitivity and may contribute to weight gain if ingested in excess. It's vital to choose good fats, such as those found in nuts, seeds, avocados, and olive oil, and to moderate intake to maintain general health.

C. Understanding Carbohydrates and Glycemic Index

The glycemic index (GI) is a measure of how quickly a carbohydrate-containing food elevates blood sugar levels. Those with a high GI are digested and absorbed swiftly, causing a rapid increase in blood glucose levels, while those with a low GI are digested and absorbed more slowly, resulting in a more gradual rise in blood sugar.

High Glycemic Foods: Examples of high GI foods are white bread, white rice, sugary cereals, and processed snacks. These foods can induce rises in blood sugar levels and should be consumed in moderation or avoided by those with diabetes.

Low Glycemic Foods: Foods with a low GI include whole grains, legumes, non-starchy vegetables, and most fruits. These foods provide a consistent amount of energy and can help regulate blood sugar levels, making them great choices for those with diabetes.

To maintain stable blood sugar levels, it's vital to focus on whole, unprocessed foods that are high in fibre and nutrients. This includes choosing whole grains over processed grains, opting for fruits and vegetables instead of sugary snacks, and balancing carbohydrate intake with protein and healthy fats.

This chapter presents an overview of diabetes types, the impact of diet on blood sugar, and the idea of glycemic index, setting the stage for the rest of the cookbook, which will focus on offering delicious dishes targeted at people managing their blood sugar levels due to diabetes

Chapter 2

Healthy Breakfast Options for Stable Blood Sugar.

Breakfast is vital for maintaining steady blood sugar levels throughout the day. In this chapter, we'll examine a selection of delicious and nutritious breakfast options designed to promote stable blood sugar levels and deliver lasting energy.

I. Understanding the Importance of Breakfast

A. Role of Breakfast in Blood Sugar Regulation:

Skipping breakfast might lead to blood sugar increases later in the day. Eating a nutritious breakfast helps manage blood sugar levels and prevents energy crashes.

B. Breakfast as a Source of Essential Nutrients:

A balanced meal includes critical nutrients such as protein, fibre, vitamins, and minerals.
Choose whole foods over processed options for maximum nourishment.

I. Low-Carb Breakfast Options

A. Egg-Based Breakfasts:

Vegetable Omelette with Spinach, Bell Peppers, and Mushrooms:

Ingredients: eggs, spinach, bell peppers, mushrooms, olive oil, salt, and pepper.

Instructions

In a bowl, mix eggs with salt and pepper.

Heat olive oil in a pan over medium heat.

Add the chopped vegetables and sauté until tender.

Pour in the beaten eggs and heat until set.

Scrambled Eggs with Avocado and **Cherry Tomatoes:**

Ingredients: eggs, avocado, cherry tomatoes, olive oil, salt, and pepper.

Instructions

Beat eggs in a basin and season with salt and pepper.

Heat olive oil in a pan over medium heat.

Add the beaten eggs and heat until scrambled.

Serve with sliced avocado and halved cherry tomatoes.

B. Greek Yogurt Parfaits

Greek Yoghourt with Berries and Almond Butter:

Ingredients:

Greek yoghurt, mixed berries, almond butter, honey.

Instructions:

Layer Greek yoghourt, mixed berries, and almond butter in a glass.
Drizzle with honey for sweetness.
Layered Greek Yogurt Parfait with Granola and Mixed Nuts:

Ingredients:
Greek yoghourt, granola, mixed nuts, honey.
Instructions:
Alternate layers of Greek yoghourt, granola, and mixed nuts in a bowl.
Drizzle with honey for added sweetness.

C. Smoothie Bowls:

Green Smoothie Bowl with Kale, Banana, and Peanut Butter:

Ingredients: kale, banana, peanut butter, almond milk, spinach, and chia seeds.

Instructions:

Blend kale, banana, peanut butter, almond milk, and spinach till smooth. Pour into a bowl and top with chia seeds.

Berry Blast Smoothie Bowl with **Mixed Berries and Coconut Flakes:**

Ingredients:

 mixed berries, coconut milk, protein powder, coconut flakes, and sliced almonds.

Instructions:

Blend the mixed berries, coconut milk, and protein powder until smooth.

Pour into a bowl and top with coconut flakes and sliced almonds.

A. Overnight Oats:

Overnight Oats with Almond Milk, Chia Seeds, and Fresh Fruit:
Ingredients: Rolled oats, almond milk, chia seeds, fresh fruit (such as berries or sliced banana), honey.
Instructions:
Mix rolled oats, almond milk, and chia seeds in a jar.
Refrigerate overnight.
In the morning, top with fresh fruit and sprinkle with honey.

Peanut Butter Banana Overnight Oats with Flax Seeds and Cinnamon:

Ingredients:
Rolled oats, almond milk, peanut butter, banana, flaxseeds, and cinnamon.

Instructions:
Combine rolled oats, almond milk, peanut butter, and mashed banana in a container.
Add flaxseeds and cinnamon.
Refrigerate overnight and enjoy in the morning.

B. Whole Grain Cereals:

Steel-Cut Oatmeal with Sliced Almonds and Berries:

Ingredients:

steel-cut oats, almond milk, sliced almonds, mixed berries, honey.

Instructions:

Cook steel-cut oats according to package instructions, using almond milk for additional smoothness.

Top with sliced almonds, mixed berries, and a drizzle of honey.

Quinoa Breakfast Bowl with Roasted Vegetables and Poached Egg:

Ingredients: cooked quinoa, roasted veggies (such as sweet potatoes, bell peppers, and zucchini), poached egg, avocado, and feta cheese.

Instructions:

Combine cooked quinoa with roasted vegetables in a bowl.

Top with a poached egg, sliced avocado, and crumbled feta cheese.

C. Nutrient-Dense Toast Toppings:

Avocado Toast with Poached Egg and Everything Bagel Seasoning:
Ingredients: whole grain bread, avocado, poached egg, and everything bagel seasoning.

Instructions:
Toast whole grain bread till golden brown.

Spread mashed avocado on the toast.

Top with a poached egg and a sprinkling of everything bagel seasoning.

Almond Butter and Banana Toast with Honey Drizzle:

Ingredients: whole grain bread, almond butter, banana, and honey.

Instructions:

Toast whole grain bread until crusty.

Spread almond butter on the toast.

Top with a sliced banana and a drizzle of honey.

IV. Balanced Breakfasts for Stable Blood Sugar

A.   Protein-Packed   Breakfast Burritos:

Whole Wheat Tortilla with Scrambled Eggs, Black Beans, and Salsa:

Ingredients: whole wheat tortilla, scrambled eggs, black beans, salsa, and avocado.

Instructions:

Fill a whole wheat tortilla with scrambled eggs, black beans, salsa, and sliced avocado.

Roll up the tortilla and enjoy.

Breakfast Burrito Bowl with Quinoa, Tofu Scramble, and Avocado:

Ingredients:

 cooked quinoa, tofu scramble, black beans, avocado, salsa.

Instructions:

Layer cooked quinoa, tofu scramble, black beans, sliced avocado, and salsa in a bowl.

Mix them together and enjoy.

B. Homemade Breakfast Muffins:

Banana Nut Muffins using Whole Wheat Flour and Oats:

Ingredients:

1 1/2 cups whole wheat flour
1 cup rolled oats
3 ripe bananas, mashed
2 big eggs
1/2 cup almond milk (or any milk of your choice)
1/2 cup chopped walnuts
1 teaspoon baking powder
1 teaspoon ground cinnamon

Instructions:

Preheat the oven: Preheat your oven to 350°F (175°C). Line a muffin tin with paper liners or coat it with cooking spray.

Mix Dry Ingredients: In a large mixing bowl, combine the whole wheat flour, rolled oats, baking powder, and ground cinnamon. Stir until well blended.

Prepare Wet Ingredients: In another basin, mash the ripe bananas with a fork until smooth. Add the eggs and almond milk to the mashed bananas and whisk together until fully mixed.

Combine Wet and Dry Ingredients: Pour the wet ingredients into the bowl containing the dry ingredients. Stir until just mixed. Be careful not to overmix.

Fold in Chopped Walnuts: Gently fold in the chopped walnuts into the muffin batter until evenly distributed.

Fill Muffin Cups: Divide the batter evenly among the prepared muffin cups, filling each about 3/4 full.

Bake: Place the muffin tray in the preheated oven and bake for 20–25 minutes, or until the muffins are golden brown and a toothpick inserted into the centre comes out clean

Cool: Remove the muffins from the oven and allow them to cool in the pan for a few minutes before transferring them to a wire rack to cool entirely.

Serve: Once chilled, serve the muffins warm or at room temperature. Enjoy them as a healthy and delicious breakfast choice!

These Banana Nut Muffins are prepared with healthy ingredients like whole wheat flour, oats, and ripe bananas, and are filled with protein and from the walnuts. They are great for a quick and tasty breakfast or snack, helping to keep your blood sugar levels steady throughout the day.

Blueberry Almond Muffins with Greek Yogurt and Lemon Zest:

Ingredients:

2 cups of almond flour
1/2 cup Greek yoghurt
3 big eggs
1 cup of fresh blueberries
1 teaspoon of almond extract
Zest of 1 lemon
1 teaspoon baking soda
1/4 cup honey (adjust to taste)

Instructions:

Preheat the oven: Preheat your oven to 350°F (175°C). Line a muffin tin with paper liners or coat it with cooking spray.

Mix Dry Ingredients: In a large mixing bowl, combine almond flour and baking soda. Stir until well blended.

Prepare Wet Ingredients: In another bowl, mix together Greek yoghurt, eggs, almond extract, lemon zest, and honey until smooth

Combine Wet and Dry Ingredients: Pour the wet ingredients into the bowl containing the dry ingredients. Stir until just mixed. Be careful not to overmix.

Fold in Blueberries: Gently fold in the fresh blueberries into the muffin batter, being careful not to crush them.

Fill Muffin Cups: Divide the batter evenly among the prepared muffin cups, filling each about 3/4 full.

Bake: Place the muffin tray in the preheated oven and bake for 20-25 minutes, or until the muffins are golden brown and a toothpick inserted into the centre comes out clean.

Cool: Remove the muffins from the oven and allow them to cool in the pan for a few minutes before transferring them to a wire rack to cool entirely.

Serve: Once chilled, serve the muffins warm or at room temperature. Enjoy them as a delicious and nutritious breakfast alternative!

These Blueberry Almond Muffins are filled with protein from the almond flour and Greek yogurt, bursting with luscious blueberries, and infused with the refreshing flavor of lemon zest. They make for a pleasant complement to any breakfast table while helping to maintain stable blood sugar levels throughout the morning.

Chapter 3

Wholesome Lunch Ideas for Sustained Energy.

Lunch isn't simply a noon meal; it's an important moment to refuel and rejuvenate for the remainder of the day. In this chapter, we'll explore a variety of nutritious and delicious lunch options designed to give sustained energy and keep you feeling satiated until supper.

I. A Balanced Plate Approach to Lunch

A. Incorporating Lean Proteins

Lean proteins are vital for muscle repair and growth and help keep you feeling full longer. Options include grilled chicken, turkey, tofu, tempeh, and legumes like lentils and chickpeas.

B. Including Complex Carbohydrates

Complex carbs are your body's primary source of energy and help maintain stable blood sugar levels. Choose healthy grains like quinoa, brown rice, and whole wheat bread, along with starchy vegetables like sweet potatoes and squash.

C. Adding Healthy Fats

Healthy fats provide long-lasting energy and enhance brain health. Include sources such as avocado, almonds, seeds, olive oil, and fatty fish like salmon and sardines.

D. Incorporating Fiber-Rich Foods

Fiber stimulates digestion and helps you feel fuller for longer. Load up on fiber-rich meals like fruits, vegetables, legumes, and whole grains to keep your digestive system happy and your energy levels constant.

II. Low-Carb Lunch Options

A. Salad Jars with Protein (Chicken, Tofu, and Beans)

Layer protein-rich items like grilled chicken, tofu, or beans with crunchy veggies, leafy greens, and a tasty vinaigrette in a mason jar for a practical and portable lunch alternative.

B. Veggie-Packed Lettuce Wraps with Hummus or Guacamole

Swap your typical wraps with lettuce leaves loaded with hummus, guacamole, or your favorite protein and veggies for a low-carb, nutrient-packed lunch.

C. Cauliflower Rice Stir-Fry with Veggies and Lean Protein

Replace rice with cauliflower rice in a stir-fry laden with colorful vegetables and lean protein for a tasty low-carb supper.

III. High-Fiber Lunch Choices

A. Quinoa Salad with Roasted Vegetables and Chickpeas

Toss cooked quinoa with roasted carrots, chickpeas, and a lemon-tahini vinaigrette for a fiber-rich lunch that's as tasty as it is nutritious.

B. Lentil Soup with Whole Grain Bread

Enjoy a hearty cup of lentil soup topped with a slice of whole grain bread for a comforting and full dinner that's filled with fiber and protein.

C. Turkey and Vegetable Wrap with Whole Wheat Tortilla

Fill a whole wheat tortilla with sliced turkey breast, crisp veggies, and a smear of hummus or avocado for a fiber-packed lunch that's excellent for on-the-go.

IV. Protein-Packed Lunches

A. Grilled Salmon with Quinoa and Steamed Broccoli

Serve grilled salmon over a bed of quinoa with a side of steamed broccoli for a protein-rich meal that's full of omega-3 fatty acids and other important elements.

B. Turkey and Quinoa Stuffed Bell Peppers

Stuff bell peppers with a blend of cooked quinoa, ground turkey, diced vegetables, and cheese for a protein-packed lunch that's as colorful as it is delicious.

V. Balanced Lunch Bowl Ideas

A. Buddha Bowl with Brown Rice, Roasted Sweet Potatoes, Avocado, and Black Beans

Build a Buddha bowl with a base of brown rice, roasted sweet potatoes, creamy avocado, black beans, and your favorite veggies for a wholesome and fulfilling lunch.
B. Mediterranean Grain Bowl with Quinoa, Falafel, Hummus, and Greek Salad

Combine quinoa, homemade falafel, hummus, Greek salad, and a splash of tzatziki sauce for a Mediterranean-inspired grain bowl that's overflowing with flavor and nutrients.

VI. Portable Lunch Options

A. Mason Jar Salads with Layers of Veggies, Protein, and Dressing

Pack a mason jar with layers of your favorite salad ingredients, including protein, veggies, greens, and dressing, for a quick and adaptable lunch alternative.

B. Bento Box Lunches with Assorted Vegetables, Cheese, Whole Grain Crackers, and Fruit

Fill a Bento box with a selection of veggies, cheese, whole grain crackers, and fruit for a balanced and portable lunch that's excellent for picnics or on-the-go.

VII. Quick and Easy Lunch Recipes

A. Veggie and Bean Quesadillas with Salsa and Greek Yogurt

Whip together veggie and bean quesadillas paired with salsa and Greek yogurt for a simple and satisfying lunch that's ready in minutes.

B. Chickpea Salad Sandwiches with Whole Grain Bread and Veggie Sticks

Mash chickpeas with Greek yogurt, lemon juice, and spices to make a delightful chickpea salad sandwich filling served on whole grain toast with veggie sticks on the side.

VIII. Tips for Meal Prep and Planning

A. Batch Cooking Protein and Grains for Easy Assembly

Spend some time on the weekend batch cooking proteins like grilled chicken and quinoa for quick and easy lunch assembly throughout the week.

B. Prepping Vegetables and Salad Ingredients Ahead of Time

Wash, chop, and store veggies ahead of time to streamline lunch prep and

make it easier to throw together a salad or stir-fry on hectic days.
C. Storing Lunches in Portion-Controlled Containers for Grab-and-Go Convenience

Invest in portion-controlled containers to portion out leftovers or packed lunches for grab-and-go ease during the week.
IX. Conclusion

Eating a good and balanced lunch is crucial to maintaining energy levels and staying productive throughout the day. By including a range of healthy nutrients and flavors in your midday meals, you may nourish your body and mind for optimal performance and well-being.

This chapter includes a complete guide to crafting healthy and delicious lunches that will keep you feeling satiated and invigorated all afternoon. Each dish and suggestion is designed to highlight nutrient-rich ingredients and balanced macronutrients to support sustained energy levels and general wellness.

Chapter 4

Nourishing Dinner Recipes to Control Blood Glucose Levels.

A. Importance of Dinner in Blood Glucose Management

Dinner has a significant role in managing blood glucose levels, especially for people with diabetes or those seeking steady energy levels.
A balanced diet during dinner helps prevent spikes and dips in blood sugar levels.
B. Focus on Nourishing Ingredients for Stable Blood Sugar Levels

Choosing nutrient-dense products ensures continuous energy and enhances overall wellness.

Recipes will contain lean proteins, fiber-rich carbs, and healthy fats for optimal blood glucose regulation.

I. Understanding the Impact of Dinner on Blood Glucose

A. Effects of Macronutrients on Blood Sugar Levels

Carbohydrates, proteins, and lipids impact blood glucose levels differently.

Consideration of the glycemic index aids in selecting foods with the minimum impact on blood sugar.

B. Timing and Portion Control for Blood Glucose Regulation

Timing meals reduces late-night blood sugar swings.
Portion control prevents excessive carbohydrate intake, which can contribute to blood sugar increases

II. Low-Glycemic Dinner Options

A. Grilled Salmon with Roasted Vegetables

Season fish with herbs and serve with roasted broccoli, cauliflower, and bell peppers.

Salmon delivers protein and omega-3 fatty acids, while vegetables supply fiber for stable blood sugar.

B. Turkey and Vegetable Stir-Fry with Brown Rice

Create a stir-fry with lean turkey, colorful vegetables, and brown rice. Turkey offers protein, vegetables add fiber, and brown rice provides complex carbs for sustained energy.

C. Lentil and Vegetable Soup with Whole Grain Bread

Prepare a hearty soup with lentils, carrots, celery, and spinach, served with whole grain bread.

Lentils and vegetables offer fiber, while whole grain bread provides carbs for steady blood sugar

III. Balanced Dinner Plate Approach

A. Incorporating Lean Proteins

Options include poultry, fish, tofu, and legumes to promote fullness and muscle health.

B. Including Fiber-Rich Carbohydrates

Incorporate whole grains, beans, and vegetables for sustained energy and digestive health.

C. Adding Healthy Fats

Avocado, nuts, seeds, and olive oil provide flavor and satiety without spiking blood sugar.

IV. Plant-Based Dinner Ideas

A. Chickpea and Spinach Curry with Quinoa

Make a flavorful curry with chickpeas, spinach, and quinoa, seasoned with aromatic spices.
Plant-based proteins and quinoa offer a balanced meal with minimal impact on blood sugar.

B. Tofu and Vegetable Skewers with Quinoa Pilaf

Skewer tofu and colorful vegetables, served with quinoa pilaf.
Tofu provides protein, vegetables add fiber, and quinoa offers complex carbs for sustained energy.

C. Roasted Vegetable and White Bean Salad

Toss roasted vegetables and white beans with fresh herbs and lemon vinaigrette.
The combination of roasted veggies and beans provides a satisfying, fiber-rich meal.

V. Dinner Recipes for Meal Prep

A. One-Pot Chicken and Vegetable Quinoa Casserole

Combine chicken, vegetables, and quinoa in a casserole dish for easy meal prep.

Batch cooking ensures convenient, balanced dinners throughout the week.

B. Stuffed Bell Peppers with Ground Turkey and Quinoa

Fill bell peppers with ground turkey, quinoa, and vegetables, topped with cheese.

Preparing ahead and baking when ready offers a nutritious, reheatable meal.

C. Sheet Pan Baked Cod with Roasted Vegetables

Bake cod with seasonal veggies on a sheet pan for a quick, easy dinner.

Minimal preparation and cleaning make this a weeknight favorite.

VI. Quick and Easy Dinner Recipes

A. Lemon Garlic Shrimp on Zucchini Noodles

Sauté shrimp with garlic and lemon, serve over zucchini noodles.
Spiralized vegetables provide a low-carb alternative to regular pasta.

B. Eggplant Parmesan with Mixed Green Salad

Bake breaded eggplant slices with marinara and cheese, serve with a mixed green salad.
A healthier rendition of a traditional dish without compromising flavor.

C. Turkey and Black Bean Tacos with Lettuce Wraps

Season ground turkey and black beans, serve in lettuce wraps with garnishes.
Lettuce wraps are a low-carb option for taco night.

VII. Tips for Dining Out and Social Gatherings

A. Making Healthier Choices at Restaurants

Navigate menus for healthier selections, and practice portion management.

Mindful selections reduce blood sugar rises while dining out.

B. Strategies for Managing Portions and Temptations

Control portions and reject unhealthy temptations in social situations. Planning ahead ensures adherence to blood sugar management targets.

Chapter 5

Snacks and Appetisers for Balanced Blood Sugar

A. Importance of Snacks and Appetisers in Blood Sugar Management

Snacks and appetisers serve a vital role in maintaining normal blood sugar levels between meals. Choosing nutrient-dense foods ensures continuous energy and reduces blood sugar spikes

.

B. Focus on Nutrient-Dense Options for Sustained Energy

Prioritising snacks and appetisers rich in protein, healthy fats, and fibre increases overall health and satiety. Understanding the glycemic index helps select foods that have a minimum impact on blood sugar levels.

I. Understanding the Role of Snacks in Blood Sugar Control

A. Effects of Snacking on Blood Glucose Levels

Snacking influences blood glucose levels and insulin responsiveness throughout the day.
Balanced foods help minimize energy crashes and cravings.

B. Strategies for Choosing Balanced Snacks

Opt for foods that mix protein, healthy fats, and fibre to decrease glucose absorption.
Practice portion control and mindful snacking to maintain blood sugar homeostasis.

II. Low-Glycemic Snack Options

A. Nut Butter and Apple Slices

Spread natural nut butter on apple slices for a pleasant and nutrient-rich snack.
Protein and fibre in nut butter ,and apples balance blood sugar levels.

B. Greek Yogurt with Berries and Almonds

Top Greek yoghurt with fresh berries and almonds for a protein-packed snack.

Greek yoghurt delivers protein and probiotics, while berries offer antioxidants, and almonds supply healthy fats.

C. Veggie Sticks with Hummus

Pair colourful veggie sticks with homemade or store-bought hummus. Fibre-rich veggies and protein-rich hummus improve satiety and blood sugar stability.

A. Caprese Skewers with Cherry Tomatoes, Mozzarella, and Basil

Skewer cherry tomatoes, fresh mozzarella, and basil, drizzle with balsamic glaze.
Protein in mozzarella and antioxidants in tomatoes and basil make this snack healthy

B. Smoked Salmon Cucumber Bites

Place smoked salmon atop cucumber slices with Greek yogurt and dill.
Omega-3 fatty acids in salmon and probiotics in yogurt boost heart and intestinal health.

Deviled Eggs with Avocado

Prepare deviled eggs with mashed avocado for a healthier option.
Protein and good fats in eggs and avocado offer balanced nourishment.

IV. Fiber-Rich Snack Ideas

A. Whole Grain Crackers with Cottage Cheese and Sliced Cucumber

Pair whole grain crackers with cottage cheese and cucumber slices.
Fiber in crackers and cucumbers, paired with protein in cottage cheese, increases blood sugar stability.

B. Edamame with Sea Salt

Steam edamame and sprinkle with sea salt for a nutritious snack.

The protein and fiber in edamame make it a good choice for blood sugar control.

C. Popcorn with Herbs and Parmesan Cheese

Season air-popped popcorn with spices and grated Parmesan cheese.

Whole grains in popcorn and protein in Parmesan cheese create a satisfying snack.

V. Quick and Easy Snacks for On-the-Go

A. Trail Mix with Nuts, Seeds, and Dried Fruit

Combine nuts, seeds, and dried fruit for a handy and energising snack. Protein, healthy fats, and fibre in trail mix provide continuous energy.

B. Hard-Boiled Eggs with Whole Grain Crackers

Pair hard-boiled eggs with whole grain crackers for a protein-packed snack. Convenience and vitamin richness make this snack excellent for busy days.

C. Protein Bars with Minimal Added Sugar

Choose protein bars with low added sugar and whole food ingredients.

Protein bars offer a convenient and healthy snack choice.

VI. Homemade Snack Recipes for Meal Prep

A. Energy Balls with Oats, Dates, and Almond Butter

Prepare energy balls with oats, dates, almond butter, and other nutritional components.

Complex carbs, protein, and healthy fats in energy balls deliver prolonged energy.

B. Roasted Chickpeas with Herbs and Spices

Season chickpeas with herbs and spices, then roast them for a crispy snack.

Protein and fibre in chickpeas make them a nutritious alternative for blood sugar management.

C. Vegetable Frittata Muffins

Make vegetable frittata muffins packed with bright veggies, eggs, and cheese.

Customizable and protein-rich, frittata muffins are perfect for meal prep.

A. Crudités Platter with Assorted Vegetables and Yogurt Dip

Assemble a crudités dish with fresh veggies served with yogurt dip.
Fiber-rich vegetables and protein-rich yogurt make this appetizer wholesome and fulfilling.

B. Stuffed Mini Peppers with Cream Cheese and Herbs

Fill tiny peppers with herbed cream cheese for a tasty snack.
Vitamin C in peppers and protein in cream cheese offer a balanced alternative.

C. Grilled Shrimp Skewers with Citrus Marinade

Prepare grilled shrimp skewers with a citrus marinade for a light and delicious appetizer.

Protein-rich shrimp and antioxidants in citrus offer a healthful option.

VIII. Tips for Snack Planning and Portion Control

A. Preparing Snacks in Advance for Convenience

Batch prepares snacks for simple grab-and-go options.

Planning beforehand ensures healthier choices throughout the day.

B. Portioning Snacks to Avoid Overeating

Portion snacks into individual servings to prevent overindulgence. Mindful portioning helps with better blood sugar regulation.

C. Incorporating Variety for Nutritional Balance

Rotate snacks to incorporate a variety of nutrients and flavors. Enjoying a varied selection of snacks ensures balanced nutrition.

IX. Conclusion

A. Recap of Key Snack and Appetiser Ideas for Balanced Blood Sugar

Summarise the relevance of selecting nutrient-dense options for blood sugar management.

Encourage experimentation with diverse flavours and ingredients.

B. Commitment to Prioritising Nutritious Snacks for Optimal Health and Wellness

Emphasise the function of snacks and appetisers in boosting general health and well-being.

Reiterate the importance of making informed decisions for sustained energy and blood sugar stability.

This chapter gives a detailed guide on selecting and cooking snacks and appetizers that encourage regulated blood sugar levels while providing delicious and gratifying options for any occasion.

Chapter 6

Desserts and Sweet Treats with Diabetic-Friendly Ingredients

A. Importance of Enjoying Desserts in Moderation

Desserts serve as a source of joy and celebration, but moderation is crucial, especially for people managing diabetes.

B. Focus on Using Diabetic-Friendly Ingredients

Diabetic-friendly components are lower in sugar and richer in fibre and healthy fats, ensuring balanced blood sugar levels and overall wellness.

I. Understanding the Impact of Desserts on Blood Sugar

A. Effects of Sugar on Blood Glucose Levels

Refined sweets can produce blood sugar spikes and insulin resistance, necessitating the need for reduced sugar consumption.

B. Strategies for Creating Diabetic-Friendly Desserts

Reducing sugar levels while retaining taste and texture by using alternative sweeteners and whole food ingredients.

II. Low-Sugar Dessert Options

A. Fruit-Based Desserts

Recipe 1: Berry Chia Jam

Ingredients:
2 cups mixed berries (strawberries, raspberries, blueberries)
2 tbsp. chia seeds
1-2 tbsp honey or maple syrup (optional)
Instructions:
In a saucepan, boil the berries over medium heat until they start to break down, stirring regularly.
Mash the berries with a fork or potato masher to desired consistency.

Stir in chia seeds and sugar, if using, and boil for another 5-10 minutes until thickened.

Remove from heat and let cool before transferring to a jar. Refrigerate for at least an hour to allow the jam to set.

B. Nut and Seed-Based Treats

Recipe 2: Almond Butter Energy Balls

Ingredients:

1 cup almond butter

1/2 cup rolled oats

1/4 cup ground flaxseed

2 tbsp honey or maple syrup

1 tsp vanilla extract

Pinch of salt

Optional add-ins: chopped nuts, seeds, dark chocolate chips

Instructions:

In a mixing bowl, add almond butter, rolled oats, ground flaxseed, honey or maple syrup, vanilla extract, and salt.

Mix until well blended. If the mixture is too dry, add a touch more almond butter or honey.

Fold in optional add-ins, if using.

Roll the mixture into small balls using your hands and place them on a baking sheet lined with parchment paper.

Chill in the refrigerator for at least 30 minutes before serving. Store leftovers in an airtight jar in the fridge.

C. Dairy-Free and Vegan Desserts

Recipe 3: Coconut Milk Popsicles

Ingredients:

1 can (14 oz) full-fat coconut milk

2 tbsp honey or maple syrup

1 tsp vanilla extract

1 cup mixed berries (strawberries, blueberries, raspberries)

Instructions:

In a blender, combine coconut milk, honey or maple syrup, and vanilla essence. Blend until smooth.

Divide mixed berries among popsicle moulds.

Pour coconut milk mixture over the fruit, filling each mould to the top.

Insert popsicle sticks and freeze for at least 4 hours or until firm.

To release popsicles, run the moulds under warm water for a few seconds. Enjoy immediately.

III. Sugar Substitutes and Alternative Sweeteners

A. Natural Sweeteners

B. Artificial Sweeteners

IV. Indulgent Dessert Recipes with a Healthy Twist

A. Chocolate Avocado Mousse

Recipe 4: Chocolate Avocado Mousse

Ingredients:
2 ripe avocados
1/4 cup cocoa powder
1/4 cup honey or maple syrup
1 tsp vanilla extract
Pinch of salt
Optional toppings: whipped coconut cream, shaved dark chocolate
Instructions:
Scoop the flesh of the avocados into a food processor or blender.
Add cocoa powder, honey or maple syrup, vanilla essence, and salt.
Blend until smooth and creamy, scraping down the sides as required.

Divide the mousse into serving dishes and refrigerate for at least 30 minutes to chill.

Serve topped with whipped coconut cream and shaved dark chocolate, if desired.

B. Berry Chia Seed Pudding

C. Almond Flour Banana Bread

V. Tips for Enjoying Desserts Mindfully

A. Portion Control and Moderation

B. Balancing Desserts with Nutrient-Dense Foods

VI. Conclusion

A. Recap of Key Points on Diabetic-Friendly Desserts

B. Commitment to Exploring New Flavours and Ingredients

This chapter includes a selection of delectable dessert options that are lower in sugar, higher in fiber and healthy fats, and mindful of blood sugar control, ensuring that those managing diabetes can still enjoy gratifying sweet treats in moderation.

Chapter 7

A. Fresh and Vibrant Salad Greens

Salad greens provide a healthful and tasty base for salads, delivering a range of textures and tastes.

B. Wholesome Salad Ingredients

Incorporating a varied range of ingredients adds depth and complexity to salads, boosting both flavour and nutrition.

I. Fresh and Vibrant Salad Greens

A. Spinach and Strawberry Salad

Ingredients:

4 cups baby spinach leaves

1 cup sliced strawberries

1/4 cup crumbled feta cheese

1/4 cup sliced almonds

Balsamic vinaigrette dressing

Instructions:

In a large bowl, add baby spinach, sliced strawberries, crumbled feta cheese, and sliced almonds.

Drizzle with balsamic vinaigrette dressing and toss lightly to coat.

Serve immediately as a refreshing and healthful salad choice.

B. Kale and Quinoa Salad

Ingredients:

4 cups chopped kale leaves

1 cup cooked quinoa

1/2 cup diced cucumber

1/2 cup cherry tomatoes, halved

1/4 cup crumbled goat cheese

Lemon tahini dressing

Instructions:

In a large bowl, massage chopped kale leaves with a touch of olive oil to soften.

Add cooked quinoa, diced cucumber, cherry tomatoes, and crumbled goat cheese to the bowl.

Drizzle with lemon tahini dressing and toss well to mix.

Allow flavours to mingle for a few minutes before serving. Enjoy this delicious and nutrient-packed salad.

II. Wholesome Salad Ingredients

A. Colourful Vegetable Medley Salad

Ingredients:

2 cups mixed salad greens

1/2 cup shredded carrots

1/2 cup sliced bell peppers (assorted hues)

1/2 cup cherry tomatoes, halved

1/4 cup chopped red onions

1/4 cup crumbled blue cheese

Red wine vinaigrette dressing

Instructions:

In a large salad bowl, blend mixed salad greens, shredded carrots, sliced bell peppers, cherry tomatoes, and sliced red onions.

Sprinkle crumbled blue cheese over the salad.

Drizzle with red wine vinaigrette dressing and stir lightly to coat all the contents.

Serve immediately as a vivid and tasty salad option.

B. Mediterranean Chickpea Salad

Ingredients:

2 cups cooked chickpeas (canned or prepared from dried)

1 cucumber, diced

1 cup cherry tomatoes, halved

1/4 cup chopped red onion

1/4 cup chopped fresh parsley

1/4 cup crumbled feta cheese

Lemon herb dressing

Instructions:

In a large mixing dish, add cooked chickpeas, sliced cucumber, cherry tomatoes, diced red onion, chopped fresh parsley, and crumbled feta cheese.

Drizzle with lemon herb dressing and toss lightly to coat all the ingredients equally.

Allow the flavours to mingle for a few minutes before serving. Enjoy this refreshing and protein-packed salad.

This chapter includes a collection of inventive and healthful salad recipes that showcase the colourful flavours and nutritious ingredients of salads, providing options for diverse tastes and preferences.

Chapter 8

One-Pot Meals for Easy Cooking and Blood Sugar Management

A. Simplicity in Cooking

One-pot meals provide a convenient solution for persons controlling blood sugar levels, minimising preparation time and cleanup.

B. Balanced Nutrition

These recipes focus on adding lean meats, whole grains, and fibre-rich veggies to support stable blood sugar levels and overall wellness.

I. One-Pot Meal Recipes

A. Quinoa and Vegetable Stir-Fry

Ingredients:

1 cup quinoa, washed

2 cups water or low-sodium vegetable broth

1 tbsp olive oil

2 cloves garlic, minced

1 onion, diced

1 bell pepper, sliced

1 cup broccoli florets

1 cup sliced mushrooms

1 cup snap peas

2 tbsp low-sodium soy sauce

Salt and pepper to taste

Instructions:

In a large pot, bring water or vegetable broth to a boil. Add quinoa, cover, and boil for 15-20 minutes, or until quinoa is cooked and water is absorbed.

In the same saucepan, heat olive oil over medium heat. Add garlic and onion, and sauté until softened.

Add bell pepper, broccoli, mushrooms, and snap peas to the pot. Cook until vegetables are tender-crisp.

Stir in cooked quinoa and soy sauce. Season with salt and pepper to taste.

Serve hot, possibly topped with chopped green onions or sesame seeds.

B. Turkey and Spinach Pasta

Ingredients:

8 oz whole wheat pasta

1 pound lean ground turkey

2 cloves garlic, minced

1 onion, diced

1 bell pepper, diced

2 cups baby spinach leaves

1 can (14.5 oz) chopped tomatoes

1 cup low-sodium chicken broth

1 tsp dry Italian seasoning

Salt and pepper to taste

Instructions:

Cook whole wheat pasta according to package instructions. Drain and set aside.

In a large pot, saute ground turkey over medium heat until browned. Add garlic and onion, and sauté until softened.

Stir in chopped bell pepper, baby spinach, diced tomatoes, chicken broth, dried Italian seasoning, salt, and pepper. Simmer for 10 minutes.

Add cooked pasta to the pot and mix to incorporate.

Serve hot, perhaps garnished with grated Parmesan cheese.

C. Salmon and Vegetable Parcel

Ingredients:

4 salmon fillets

2 tbsp lemon juice

2 tbsp olive oil

2 cloves garlic, minced

1 tsp dried dill

1 zucchini, sliced

1 yellow squash, sliced

1 bell pepper, sliced

1 cup cherry tomatoes

Salt and pepper to taste

Instructions:

Preheat the oven to 375°F (190°C). Cut four large pieces of parchment paper.

In a small bowl, mix lemon juice, olive oil, minced garlic, dried dill, salt, and pepper.

Place a salmon fillet on each piece of parchment paper. Season with salt and pepper, then drizzle with the lemon juice mixture.

Arrange sliced zucchini, yellow squash, bell pepper, and cherry tomatoes around each salmon fillet.

Fold the parchment paper over the salmon and vegetables to make a bundle, sealing the sides tightly.

Place packages on a baking sheet and bake in the warmed oven for 15-20 minutes, or until fish is cooked through and veggies are tender.

Serve hot, optionally garnished with fresh herbs like parsley or dill.

II. Conclusion

A. Embracing One-Pot Meals

Incorporating these simple and nutritious one-pot dishes into your meal plan helps expedite cooking while supporting stable blood sugar levels.

B. Experiment and Enjoy

Feel free to alter these recipes using your favorite ingredients and tastes to fit your taste preferences and dietary restrictions.

This chapter presents a range of delicious and easy-to-make one-pot meals that are great for persons controlling blood sugar level

Chapter 9

Quick and Easy Meals for Busy Days

Living a busy lifestyle typically means limited time for food preparation. In this chapter, we'll explore a number of quick and easy meal choices designed to fit into even the busiest of schedules. From breakfast to dinner and everything in between, these recipes and methods will help you nourish yourself and your family without sacrificing taste or nutrition.

Section 1: Breakfast Solutions

1.1 Grab-and-Go Breakfasts

Homemade Breakfast Bars:

Ingredients:
2 cups rolled oats
1 cup nuts or seeds (e.g., almonds, pumpkin seeds)
1 cup dried fruit (e.g., raisins, dried cranberries)
1/2 cup honey or maple syrup
1/4 cup nut butter (e.g., almond butter, peanut butter)
1 tsp vanilla extract
Instructions:
In a large bowl, mix together oats, nuts or seeds, and dried fruit.

In a small saucepan, simmer honey or maple syrup, nut butter, and vanilla extract over low heat until melted and mixed.

Pour the wet components over the dry ingredients and whisk until evenly coated.

Press the mixture into a prepared baking dish and chill for at least 2 hours.

Cut into bars and keep in an airtight container for up to one week.

Make-Ahead Breakfast Burritos:

Ingredients:

6 big eggs

1/4 cup milk

Salt and pepper to taste

6 large flour tortillas or whole wheat wraps

1 cup cooked black beans

1 cup cooked quinoa

1 cup shredded cheese

Salsa, avocado, or additional toppings of choice

Instructions:

In a large bowl, whisk together eggs, milk, salt, and pepper.

In a skillet, scramble the eggs until cooked through.

Lay out tortillas and divide scrambled eggs, black beans, quinoa, and cheese among them.

Roll up the tortillas, folding in the sides, to form burritos.

Wrap each burrito firmly in aluminum foil and store in the refrigerator or freezer.

To reheat, remove foil and microwave on high for 1-2 minutes (if refrigerated) or 3-4 minutes (if frozen).

Section 2: Lunchtime Solutions

2.1 Portable Lunches

Turkey and Avocado Wrap:

Ingredients:

4 large whole wheat wraps

1 pound sliced turkey breast

1 avocado, sliced

1 cup spinach leaves

1/2 cup shredded cheese

1/4 cup ranch dressing or mayonnaise

Instructions:

Lay out wraps and divide turkey, avocado, spinach, and cheese evenly among them.

Drizzle with ranch dressing or spread with mayonnaise.

Roll up the wraps tightly, tucking in the sides, to form burritos.

Cut in half and wrap firmly in aluminum foil or plastic wrap for convenient transport.

2.2 No-Cook Lunches

Greek Chickpea Salad:

Ingredients:

2 cans (15 oz each) chickpeas, drained and rinsed

1 cucumber, diced

1 bell pepper, diced

1 cup cherry tomatoes, halved

1/2 cup crumbled feta cheese

1/4 cup chopped fresh parsley

1/4 cup olive oil

2 tbsp lemon juice

1 tsp dried oregano

Salt and pepper to taste

Instructions:

In a large bowl, add chickpeas, cucumber, bell pepper, tomatoes, feta cheese, and parsley.

In a small bowl, whisk together olive oil, lemon juice, oregano, salt, and pepper.

Pour the dressing over the salad and toss until evenly coated.

Divide into individual containers and chill until ready to eat.

Section 3: Dinner in a Flash

3.1 One-Pot Wonders

One-Pot Pasta Primavera:

Ingredients:
8 oz pasta (penne or spaghetti)
2 cups chopped vegetables (e.g., bell peppers, zucchini, cherry tomatoes)
2 cloves garlic, minced
4 cups vegetable broth
1/2 cup grated Parmesan cheese
2 tbsp olive oil
Salt and pepper to taste

Instructions:

In a large pot, add pasta, veggies, garlic, and vegetable broth.

Bring to a boil over medium-high heat, then lower to a simmer and cook until pasta is al dente and vegetables are cooked, stirring periodically.

Stir in Parmesan cheese and olive oil until melted and thoroughly blended.

Season with salt and pepper to taste before serving.

3.2 Sheet Pan Suppers

Sheet Pan Chicken with Vegetables:

Ingredients:

4 boneless, skinless chicken breasts
2 cups broccoli florets

2 cups baby carrots

1 cup cherry tomatoes

2 tbsp olive oil

1 tsp garlic powder

1 tsp Italian seasoning

Salt and pepper to taste

Instructions:

Preheat the oven to 400°F (200°C). Line a baking sheet with parchment paper.

Place chicken breasts on one side of the baking sheet and arrange vegetables on the other half.

Drizzle olive oil over chicken and vegetables, then sprinkle with garlic powder, Italian seasoning, salt, and pepper.

Bake for 20-25 minutes, or until chicken is cooked through and vegetables are soft.
Section 4: Snack Attack

4.1 Healthy Snack Ideas

Apple Slices with Peanut Butter:

Ingredients:
2 apples, cut
1/4 cup peanut butter
Instructions:
Arrange apple slices on a dish or serving platter.
Serve with peanut butter for dipping.

4.2 Energy Boosting Snacks

Trail Mix:

Ingredients:

1 cup mixed nuts (e.g., almonds, cashews, walnuts)

1/2 cup dried fruit (e.g., raisins, cranberries, apricots)

1/4 cup dark chocolate chips or chunks

1/4 cup pumpkin seeds

Instructions:

In a large bowl, add nuts, dried fruit, dark chocolate chips or chunks, and pumpkin seeds.

Mix carefully to evenly distribute the ingredients.

Store in an airtight container for a handy energy-boosting snack on the run. Enjoy!

Chapter 10

Family-Friendly Recipes the Whole Household Will Love.

Desserts are the perfect way to end a family supper on a sweet note. Whether it's a big event or just a typical day, these wonderful delicacies are sure to please everyone in the household.

A. Fresh Fruit Skewers with Yogurt Dip

Ingredients:

Assorted fresh fruits (strawberries, pineapple, grapes, kiwi, melon)
Greek yoghourt (simple or flavoured)
Honey (optional, for sweetening yoghourt)
Bamboo skewers or cocktail sticks
Instructions:

Wash and prepare the fruits by cutting them into bite-sized pieces.

Thread the fruit pieces onto bamboo skewers or cocktail sticks, alternating different fruits for variety.

In a small bowl, mix the Greek yoghourt with honey if desired, to sweeten.

Serve the fruit skewers with the bowl of yoghourt dip on the side for dipping.

B. Homemade Cookies or Brownies

Ingredients:

1 cup (2 sticks) unsalted butter, softened

1 cup granulated sugar

1 cup packed brown sugar

2 big eggs

1 teaspoon vanilla extract

2 1/4 cups all-purpose flour

1 teaspoon baking soda

1/2 teaspoon salt

2 cups semisweet chocolate chips (for cookies) or 1 cup cocoa powder (for brownies)

Optional mix-ins: chopped nuts, dried fruit, candies

Instructions:

Preheat the oven to 375°F (190°C) for cookies or 350°F (175°C) for brownies. Grease a baking sheet or line it with parchment paper.

In a large mixing bowl, cream together the softened butter, granulated sugar, and brown sugar until light and fluffy.

Beat in the eggs, one at a time, then stir in the vanilla extract.

In a separate bowl, whisk together the flour, baking soda, and salt. Gradually add the dry ingredients to the wet ingredients, mixing until well combined.

If making cookies, fold in the chocolate chips or other mix-ins of your choice. If making brownies, mix in the cocoa powder until fully incorporated.

Drop spoonfuls of cookie dough onto the prepared baking sheet, spacing them about 2 inches apart, or spread the brownie batter evenly into the prepared baking pan.

Bake cookies for 8-10 minutes or until golden brown around the edges.

Bake brownies for 25-30 minutes or until a toothpick inserted into the centre comes out clean.

Allow the cookies or brownies to cool slightly before transferring them to a wire rack to cool completely.

C. Frozen Banana Pops

Ingredients:

Ripe bananas

Wooden popsicle sticks or skewers
Semisweet chocolate chips or melting
chocolate
Chopped nuts, sprinkles, crushed
coconut (optional garnishes)

Instructions:
Peel the bananas and split them in
half crosswise. Insert a wooden
popsicle stick or skewer into the cut
end of each banana half.
Place the bananas on a
parchment-lined baking sheet and
freeze for at least 1 hour until hard.
Melt the chocolate chips or melted
chocolate in a microwave-safe basin
according to package instructions,
stirring until smooth.

Dip each frozen banana into the melting chocolate, using a spoon to help coat it evenly. Allow any excess chocolate to fall off.

Sprinkle the chocolate-coated bananas with chopped nuts, sprinkles, shredded coconut, or any other desired toppings.

Place the covered bananas back onto the parchment-lined baking sheet and return them to the freezer until the chocolate sets, about 15-20 minutes.

Once the chocolate is solid, the frozen banana pops are ready to enjoy. Store any leftovers in an airtight jar in the freezer.

Enjoy these dessert pleasures with your family for a delicious and sweet finale to your meals!

Chapter 11

Low-Carb and Keto-Friendly Recipes for Blood Sugar Control

Dessert can still be pleasant while sticking to a low-carb or keto lifestyle. These dessert recipes are not only delicious but also assist in maintaining stable blood sugar levels, making them excellent options for anyone wanting to control their blood sugar.

A. Sugar-Free Cheesecake Bites

Traditional cheesecake is generally filled with sugar and carbohydrates, but these sugar-free cheesecake bites offer a delightful alternative. By utilising sugar replacements and almond flour, these pieces are low in carbohydrates while yet giving the creamy richness of cheesecake.

Ingredients:

8 oz cream cheese, softened
1/2 cup almond flour
1/4 cup powdered stevia or erythritol
1 tsp vanilla extract
Instructions:

In a mixing bowl, add softened cream cheese, almond flour, powdered stevia or erythritol, and vanilla essence.
Mix until well blended and smooth.

Roll the mixture into bite-sized balls and lay them on a parchment-lined baking sheet.

Chill the cheesecake pieces in the refrigerator for at least 1 hour until firm.

Serve chilled and enjoy as a guilt-free dessert.

B. Dark Chocolate Avocado Mousse

This luscious mousse gets its creamy texture from ripe avocados instead of heavy cream, making it a keto-friendly dessert option. The use of unsweetened cocoa powder and a sugar replacement delivers rich chocolate flavour without the extra sugars.

Ingredients:

2 ripe avocados
1/4 cup unsweetened cocoa powder
1/4 cup almond milk
1/4 cup powdered stevia or erythritol
1 tsp vanilla extract

Instructions:

Scoop the flesh of the avocados into a food processor or blender.

Add cocoa powder, almond milk, powdered stevia or erythritol, and vanilla extract to the avocados.

Blend until smooth and creamy, scraping down the sides as required.

Taste and adjust sweetness if necessary by adding more sweetener.

Transfer the mousse into serving dishes or glasses.

Chill in the refrigerator for at least 30 minutes before serving.

Garnish with grated dark chocolate or a dollop of whipped cream if preferred.

C. Berry Chia Seed Pudding

Chia seed pudding is a nutritious and adaptable dessert that can be modified with numerous toppings. This recipe blends chia seeds with unsweetened almond milk and mixed berries for a low-carb and keto-friendly dessert.

Ingredients:

1/4 cup chia seeds

1 cup unsweetened almond milk

1 cup mixed berries (strawberries, blueberries, raspberries)

2 tbsp powdered stevia or erythritol

Instructions:

In a mixing dish, blend chia seeds and unsweetened almond milk.

Stir thoroughly to blend and let sit for 5 minutes.

Stir again to break up any clumps of chia seeds.

Cover the bowl and refrigerate for at least 2 hours or overnight until the mixture thickens into a pudding-like consistency.

In another bowl, stir mixed berries with powdered stevia or erythritol to sweeten.

To serve, arrange the chia seed pudding and sweetened fruit in glasses or jars.

Garnish with extra berries on top if desired.

Enjoy chilled as a pleasant and nutritious dessert alternative.

These dessert delicacies offer a wonderful solution to fulfil your sweet desires while following a low-carb or keto-friendly diet. Enjoy them as part of your balanced meal plan for blood sugar control and overall well-being.

Chapter 12

Heart-Healthy Recipes for Diabetic Cardiac Health

Dessert Treats

Indulging in dessert doesn't have to sacrifice heart health or blood sugar control. These tasty dessert dishes are specifically designed to be heart-healthy and suitable for persons managing diabetes.

A. Dark Chocolate-Dipped Strawberries

Dark chocolate contains flavonoids, which have been connected with heart health benefits, while strawberries give antioxidants and fibre. This combination makes dark chocolate-dipped strawberries a nutritious and enjoyable dessert option.

Ingredients:
Fresh strawberries
Dark chocolate (70% cocoa content or greater)

Instructions:
Wash and dry the strawberries completely, leaving the stems intact.
In a microwave-safe bowl, melt the dark chocolate in 30-second intervals, stirring in between until smooth.
Dip each strawberry into the melted chocolate, coating it halfway.

Place the coated strawberries on a parchment-lined baking sheet.
Refrigerate for 15-20 minutes or until the chocolate hardens.
Serve and savour these luscious dark chocolate-dipped strawberries as a heart-healthy dessert.

B. Baked Cinnamon Apples with Greek Yoghourt

Apples are rich in fibre and antioxidants, while cinnamon may help manage blood sugar levels. Greek Yogurt provides nutrition and smoothness to this cosy treat.

Ingredients:
Apples (such as Granny Smith or Honeycrisp)

Ground cinnamon

Greek yoghourt (simple or flavoured)

Instructions:

Preheat the oven to 375°F (190°C).

Core the apples and slice them into wedges or rings.

Arrange the apple slices in a baking dish.

Sprinkle cinnamon generously over the apple pieces.

Bake for 20-25 minutes or until the apples are soft.

Serve heated with a dollop of Greek yoghourt on top.

C. Chia Seed Pudding with Mixed Berries

Chia seeds are abundant in fibre and omega-3 fatty acids, making them a healthful complement to any diet. Combined with mixed berries, this pudding is a tasty and heart-healthy dessert option

Ingredients

Chia seeds

Unsweetened almond milk

Mixed berries (such as strawberries, blueberries, raspberries)

Vanilla extract

Honey or stevia (optional, for sweetness)

Instructions:

In a dish, mix together chia seeds and almond milk in a 1:4 ratio (e.g., 1/4 cup chia seeds to 1 cup almond milk).

Add vanilla extract and sweetener if preferred.

Stir well and let it settle for 10 minutes.

Stir again to break up any clumps.

Cover and refrigerate for at least 2 hours or overnight.

Serve chilled with mixed berries on top.

These dessert options are not only delicious but also improve heart health and blood sugar control, making them great for persons managing diabetes. Enjoy them as part of a balanced diet for general well-being.

Chapter 13

Gluten-Free and Dairy-Free Options for Diabetic Diets

Living with diabetes needs careful monitoring of nutrition, and for individuals with allergies to gluten and dairy, finding adequate meal alternatives can be problematic. However, with the correct products and recipes, it's possible to have tasty and nutritious meals that are both gluten-free and dairy-free. In this chapter, we'll examine a variety of delectable foods adapted to fit the needs of those with diabetes who follow a gluten-free and dairy-free diet.

I. Introduction to Gluten-Free and Dairy-Free Eating for Diabetes Management

A. Explanation of gluten-free and dairy-free diets

1. A gluten-free diet excludes gluten, a protein found in wheat, barley, and rye, suitable for individuals with celiac disease or gluten sensitivity.

2. A dairy-free diet eliminates all dairy products, including milk,

cheese, yoghourt, and butter, commonly chosen by individuals with lactose intolerance or dairy allergies.

B. Importance of dietary modifications for individuals with diabetes

1. Diet has a critical role in maintaining blood sugar levels and general health for those with diabetes.

2. Gluten-free and dairy-free foods can assist individuals with diabetes better manage their disease and lessen symptoms associated with gluten or dairy intolerance.

C. Overview of the benefits of gluten-free and dairy-free nutrition for diabetes control

1. Reducing gluten and dairy consumption can lead to improved digestion, less inflammation, and better blood sugar control for those with diabetes.

2. Choosing nutrient-dense and balanced gluten-free and dairy-free alternatives is vital for promoting overall health and well-being.

A. Quinoa Breakfast Bowl with Fresh Fruit

1. Ingredients:

- 1/2 cup quinoa

- Assorted fresh fruit (such as berries, banana)

- 1/4 cup almond milk

- 2 tablespoons nuts or seeds (such as almonds, chia seeds)

2. Instructions:

- Rinse quinoa in cold water, then cook according to package instructions.

- Once cooked, transfer quinoa to a bowl and top with fresh fruit.

- Drizzle almond milk over the fruit and sprinkle with nuts or seeds for extra crunch.

B. Avocado Toast with Gluten-Free Bread

Ingredients:

- 2 slices gluten-free bread

- 1 ripe avocado

- 1 tablespoon lemon juice

- Salt and pepper to taste

Instructions:

- Toast the gluten-free bread till golden brown.

- Mash the ripe avocado with lemon juice, salt, and pepper.

- Spread the mashed avocado onto the toasted gluten-free bread.

III. Lunch Options

A. Gluten-Free Pasta Salad with Grilled Vegetables

1. Ingredients:

- 8 oz gluten-free spaghetti

- Assorted grilled vegetables (such as zucchini, bell peppers)

- 2 tablespoons olive oil

- 1 tablespoon balsamic vinegar

- Fresh herbs (such as basil, parsley), for garnish

Instructions:

- Cook gluten-free pasta according to package instructions, then drain and rinse with cool water.

- Grill different vegetables until soft and slightly browned, then slice into bite-sized pieces.

- In a large bowl, combine cooked pasta and grilled vegetables. Drizzle with olive oil and balsamic vinegar, then toss to coat.

- Garnish with fresh herbs before serving.

B. Dairy-Free Lentil Soup

Ingredients:

- 1 cup dried lentils

- Assorted veggies (such as carrots, celery, onions)

- 4 cups vegetable broth

- 2 cloves garlic, minced

- 1 teaspoon ground cumin

- Salt and pepper to taste

Instructions:

- Rinse lentils in cold water, then place them in a big pot with vegetable broth.

- Chop diverse vegetables and add them to the saucepan with lentils.

- Stir in minced garlic, ground cumin, salt, and pepper.

- Bring the mixture to a boil, then reduce heat and simmer for 20-25 minutes or until lentils and vegetables are cooked.

IV. Dinner Recipes

A. Baked Salmon with Roasted Potatoes and Asparagus

. **Ingredients**:

- 4 salmon fillets

- 1 pound baby potatoes, halved

- 1 bunch asparagus, trimmed

- 2 tablespoons olive oil

- 1 lemon, sliced

- 2 cloves garlic, minced

- Fresh dill, for garnish

Instructions:

- Preheat the oven to 400°F (200°C). Place salmon fillets on a baking pan lined with parchment paper.

- In a bowl, combine halved baby potatoes and trimmed asparagus with olive oil, chopped garlic, salt, and pepper. Arrange them around the salmon on the baking sheet.

- Place lemon slices on top of each salmon fillet.

- Bake in the preheated oven for 12-15 minutes, or until the salmon is cooked through and the vegetables are soft.

- Garnish with fresh dill before serving.

B. Gluten-Free and Dairy-Free Stir-Fry with Tofu and Vegetables

1. Ingredients:

- 14 oz firm tofu, squeezed and cubed

- Assorted vegetables (such as broccoli, bell peppers, snap peas)

- 3 tablespoons gluten-free soy sauce

- 2 cloves garlic, minced

- 1 tablespoon fresh ginger, grated

- 2 teaspoons sesame oil

Instructions:

- Heat sesame oil in a large skillet or wok over medium-high heat.

- Add cubed tofu to the skillet and cook until golden brown on all sides.

- Stir in minced garlic and grated ginger, then add mixed vegetables to the skillet.

- Cook until vegetables are tender-crisp, then whisk in gluten-free soy sauce.

- Serve stir-fry hot over cooked rice or quinoa.

V. Snack Ideas

A. Gluten-Free and Dairy-Free Energy Bites

. **Ingredients**:

- 1 cup gluten-free rolled oats
- 1/2 cup almond butter

- 1/4 cup honey or maple syrup

- 2 teaspoons chia seeds

- 2 teaspoons shredded coconut

Instructions:

- In a mixing dish, add rolled oats, almond butter, honey or maple syrup, chia seeds, and shredded coconut.

- Mix until well blended, then roll mixture into bite-sized balls.

- Place energy bites on a baking sheet lined with parchment paper and refrigerate for 30 minutes to solidify.

B. Veggie Sticks with Hummus

Ingredients:

- Assorted raw veggies (such as carrots, cucumbers, bell peppers)

- Store-bought or homemade hummus

Instructions:

- Wash and cut raw vegetables into sticks.

- Serve with hummus for dipping.

Chapter 14

International Flavours: Ethnic Recipes Adapted for Diabetes

A. Explanation of the notion of modifying ethnic foods for diabetes:

- Ethnic dishes can contain components high in carbs, sweets, or harmful fats, problematic for those with diabetes.

- Adapting these recipes can make them healthier and more diabetes-friendly while keeping traditional flavours.

B. Importance of cultural diversity in gastronomy and the necessity for diabetic-friendly options:

- Cultural diversity enriches culinary traditions, but those with diabetes need access to adequate options.

- Offering various, tasty, and diabetes-friendly meals improves commitment to healthy eating.

C. Overview of the benefits of introducing international tastes into diabetic diets:

- Diverse diets containing fruits, vegetables, lean proteins, and whole grains give health benefits.

- Enjoying international flavours makes diabetes meal planning enjoyable and diversified.

I. Asian Cuisine

A. Stir-Fried Tofu with Vegetables:

- Ingredients:

- 1 brick tofu, cubed

- Assorted vegetables (bell peppers, broccoli, carrots)

- 2 tbsp soy sauce

- 1 tbsp sesame oil

- 1 tbsp minced garlic

- 1 tsp grated ginger

- **Instructions:**

1. Heat sesame oil in a pan, add garlic and ginger, stir-fry for 1 minute.

2. Add tofu cubes and fry till golden brown.

3. Add vegetables and soy sauce, stir-fry until vegetables are tender.

B. Chicken and Vegetable Curry:

- **Ingredients**:

- 1 lb chicken breast, diced

- Assorted vegetables (zucchini, bell peppers, onions)

- 2 tbsp curry powder

- 1 cup coconut milk (light)

- 1 tbsp olive oil

- **Instructions**:

1. Heat olive oil in a pot, add chicken and cook until browned.

2. Add vegetables and curry powder, simmer until vegetables are tender.

3. Pour in coconut milk, boil for 10 minutes.

C. Brown Rice Sushi Rolls:

- **Ingredients**:

- 2 cups cooked brown rice

- Nori seaweed sheets

-       Assorted   fillings   (avocado, cucumber, cooked shrimp)

- Soy sauce (low-sodium)

- **Instructions**:

1. Place a sheet of nori on a bamboo sushi mat, spread a layer of brown rice.

2. Add ingredients, roll tightly, then slice into sushi rolls.

3. Serve with low-sodium soy sauce for dipping.

II. Mediterranean Cuisine

A. Grilled Mediterranean Chicken Skewers:

- **Ingredients**:

- 1 lb chicken breast, cubed

- Assorted vegetables (cherry tomatoes, bell peppers, red onions)

- 2 tbsp olive oil

- 1 tsp dried oregano

- 1 lemon, juiced

- **Instructions**:1. In a bowl, marinate chicken in olive oil, oregano, and lemon juice for 30 minutes.

2. Thread chicken and vegetables onto skewers, heat until cooked through.

B. Quinoa Tabbouleh Salad:

- **Ingredients**:

- 1 cup cooked quinoa

- Assorted vegetables (cucumber, tomatoes, parsley, mint)

- 2 tbsp lemon juice

- 1 tbsp olive oil

- Salt and pepper to taste

- **Instructions**:

1. In a bowl, add cooked quinoa and chopped vegetables.

2. Dress with lemon juice, olive oil, salt, and pepper, toss to mix.

C. Eggplant Involtini:

- **Ingredients**:

- 1 large eggplant, sliced lengthwise

- 1 cup firm tofu, mashed

- 1 cup marinara sauce (low-sugar)

- 1/4 cup nutritional yeast

- **Instructions**:

1. Grill eggplant slices till cooked, put aside.

2. Mix mashed tofu and nutritional yeast, apply onto eggplant pieces.

3. Roll up eggplant slices, lay in a baking dish, cover with marinara sauce, and bake until heated through.

Chapter 15

Comfort Foods Made Diabetic-Friendly

What is Comfort Foods and Their Significance:

Comfort foods are familiar recipes that bring emotional gratification and a sense of well-being.

They are typically associated with nostalgia and might bring solace during times of stress or nostalgia.

B. Challenges Posed by Traditional Comfort Foods for Individuals with Diabetes:

Many classic comfort meals are heavy in carbohydrates, sugars, and harmful fats, which can raise blood sugar levels and cause issues for those with diabetes.

C. Purpose of the Chapter: Providing Diabetic-Friendly Alternatives to Classic Comfort Foods:

The chapter tries to give diabetic-friendly alternatives of classic comfort foods that are reduced in carbs, sugars, and harmful fats while still being delicious and gratifying.

Breakfast Comfort Foods

A. Oatmeal with Fresh Berries and Nuts:

Description: A warm cup of oatmeal cooked with rolled oats, topped with fresh berries for natural sweetness and almonds for additional crunch and healthy fats.

Ingredients:

1/2 cup rolled oats

1 cup water or almond milk

Fresh berries (such as strawberries, blueberries, raspberries)

2 tablespoons chopped nuts (such as almonds, walnuts, pecans)

Instructions:

In a small saucepan, bring water or almond milk to a boil.

Stir in rolled oats and decrease heat to low. Cook for 5-7 minutes, stirring occasionally, until the oats are soft and the mixture thickens.

Remove from heat and allow to settle for a minute to thicken further.

Transfer oats to a bowl and top with fresh berries and chopped nuts.

Serve hot and enjoy!

B. Whole Wheat Pancakes with Sugar-Free Syrup:

Fluffy whole wheat pancakes baked with whole grain flour, served with sugar-free syrup or fruit compote for a guilt-free treat.

Ingredients:

1 cup whole wheat flour

1 tablespoon baking powder

1 tablespoon sugar replacement (such as stevia or erythritol)

1 cup almond milk (or other milk of choice)

1 egg

1 teaspoon vanilla extract

Cooking spray or coconut oil for coating the pan

Sugar-free syrup or fruit compote for serving

Instructions:

In a mixing bowl, whisk together whole wheat flour, baking powder, and sugar substitute.

In a separate bowl, whisk together almond milk, egg, and vanilla extract until well combined.

Pour wet ingredients into dry ingredients and stir until just combined. Do not overmix; the batter may be a little lumpy.

Heat a non-stick skillet or griddle over medium heat and lightly coat with cooking spray or coconut oil.

Pour 1/4 cup of batter into the griddle for each pancake. Cook until bubbles appear on the surface, then flip and cook until golden brown on the other side.

Repeat with remaining batter, coating the skillet as needed.

Serve heated pancakes with sugar-free syrup or fruit compote on top.

Enjoy your tasty and diabetic-friendly breakfast!

C. Veggie Omelette with Whole Grain Toast:

A delightful vegetarian omelette loaded with bright vegetables and served on whole grain toast for a balanced and hearty breakfast.

Ingredients:

2 eggs

1/4 cup chopped veggies (such as bell peppers, onions, spinach, tomatoes)

Salt and pepper to taste

1 teaspoon olive oil or cooking spray

1 piece whole grain bread

Instructions: In a bowl, mix together eggs until fully beaten. Season with salt and pepper.

Heat olive oil or cooking spray in a non-stick skillet over medium heat.

Add chopped vegetables to the skillet and heat until softened, about 2-3 minutes.

Pour beaten eggs over the vegetables and swirl the skillet to spread evenly.

Cook for 2-3 minutes, raising the edges with a spatula to enable raw eggs to pour below.

Once the omelette is set but still somewhat runny on top, fold it in half with the spatula.

Cook for another minute until totally set and gently browned on the bottom.

Slide the omelette onto a platter and serve with whole grain toast on the side.

Enjoy your wholesome and tasty vegetarian omelette breakfast!

Chapter 16

Seasonal Recipes: Fresh Produce and Festive Flavours

A. Explanation of Seasonal Cooking:

Seasonal cuisine emphasises using fresh, locally available items that are in season.

Benefits include better flavour, nutrition, and sustainability.

B. Celebration of Fresh Produce and Festive Flavours:

Highlighting the abundance of seasonal fruits, vegetables, and herbs.

Acknowledgment of various flavours and culinary traditions linked with different seasons and festive occasions.

C. Purpose of the Chapter:

To highlight seasonal recipes that feature the finest of each season's crops and joyful flavours.

Inspire readers to embrace seasonal cooking and enjoy the freshest ingredients year-round.

I. Spring Recipes

A. Spring Vegetable Frittata:

Light and fluffy frittata with spring vegetables like asparagus, peas, and baby spinach.

Ingredients:

6 eggs

1/4 cup milk

1 cup chopped spring vegetables

Salt and pepper to taste

Instructions:

Preheat the oven to 350°F (175°C).

Whisk eggs and milk together in a bowl. Season with salt and pepper.

Sauté veggies till tender.

Pour egg mixture over vegetables in an oven-safe skillet.

Bake for 15-20 minutes until set.

Serve hot or cold.

B. Strawberry Spinach Salad with Balsamic Vinaigrette:

Refreshing salad with fresh strawberries, baby spinach, toasted almonds, and balsamic vinaigrette.

Ingredients:

4 cups baby spinach

1 cup sliced strawberries

1/4 cup sliced almonds, toasted

2 tablespoons balsamic vinegar

1 tablespoon olive oil

1 teaspoon honey

Instructions:

In a large bowl, combine spinach, strawberries, and almonds.

In a small bowl, whisk together balsamic vinegar, olive oil, and honey.

Drizzle dressing over salad and toss to coat.

Serve immediately.

C. Lemon Herb Roasted Chicken:

 Juicy roasted chicken flavored with lemon and herbs including rosemary, thyme, and parsley.

Ingredients:

4 chicken breasts

2 lemons, sliced

2 tablespoons olive oil

2 cloves garlic, minced

1 tablespoon chopped fresh herbs (rosemary, thyme, parsley)

Instructions:

Preheat the oven to 375°F (190°C).

Rub chicken breasts with olive oil, minced garlic, and chopped herbs.

Place lemon slices on top of chicken.

Roast for 25-30 minutes until cooked through.

Serve with roasted veggies.

II. Summer Recipes

A. Grilled Vegetable Skewers with Chimichurri Sauce:

Colourful vegetable skewers cooked and served with chimichurri sauce.

Ingredients:

Assorted vegetables (bell peppers, zucchini, cherry tomatoes, mushrooms)

Wooden skewers, soaking in water

Chimichurri sauce (parsley, cilantro, garlic, olive oil, vinegar)

Instructions:

Thread vegetables onto skewers.

Grill over medium-high heat for 8-10 minutes, rotating occasionally.

Serve with chimichurri sauce.

B. Watermelon Feta Salad with Mint:

Refreshing salad with watermelon, feta cheese, mint, and balsamic sauce.

Ingredients:

4 cups cubed watermelon

1 cup crumbled feta cheese

Fresh mint leaves

Balsamic glaze

Instructions:

Arrange watermelon cubes on a serving plate.

Sprinkle it with crumbled feta cheese and torn mint leaves.

Drizzle with balsamic glaze.

Serve cold.

C. Grilled Salmon with Mango Salsa:

Grilled salmon fillets topped with fresh mango salsa.

Ingredients:

4 salmon fillets

1 mango, diced

1/4 cup chopped red onion

1/4 cup chopped cilantro

Juice of 1 lime

Salt and pepper to taste

Instructions:

Season salmon fillets with salt and pepper.

Grill over medium heat for 4-5 minutes per side.

In a bowl, add chopped mango, red onion, cilantro, and lime juice.

Spoon mango salsa over cooked fish.

Chapter 17

Slow Cooker and Instant Pot Recipes for Convenient Cooking

Slow cookers and Instant Pots have transformed food preparation, giving ease, adaptability, and tasty results with no effort. In this chapter, we'll explore a range of delectable dishes customised for these practical cooking machines, from rich stews to tender meats and nourishing soups.

I. Slow Cooker Recipes

A. Slow Cooker Beef Stew

A warm bowl of beef stew, cooked low and slow to perfection, with soft bits of beef, potatoes, carrots, and onions.

Ingredients:

2 pounds beef stew meat, cubed

4 potatoes, peeled and diced

3 carrots, sliced

1 onion, chopped

3 cloves garlic, minced

4 cups beef broth

2 tablespoons tomato paste

1 teaspoon Worcestershire sauce

1 teaspoon dried thyme

Salt and pepper to taste

Instructions:

Place beef stew meat, potatoes, carrots, onion, and garlic in the slow cooker.

In a bowl, whisk together beef broth, tomato paste, Worcestershire sauce, thyme, salt, and pepper. Pour over the steak and vegetables.

Cover and simmer on low for 8 hours or on high for 4 hours until beef is tender.

Serve hot, garnished with fresh parsley if preferred.

B. Crockpot Chicken Tikka Masala

A tasty Indian-inspired dish containing delicate chicken cooked in a creamy tomato-based sauce with aromatic spices.

Ingredients:

1.5 pounds boneless, skinless chicken breasts, cut into cubes

1 onion, finely chopped

3 cloves garlic, minced

1 tablespoon ginger, grated

1 can (14 oz) chopped tomatoes

1 cup coconut milk

2 tablespoons tomato paste

2 teaspoons garam masala

1 teaspoon ground cumin

1 teaspoon ground coriander

1/2 teaspoon turmeric

Salt and pepper to taste

Fresh cilantro for garnish

Instructions:

Place chicken, onion, garlic, ginger, diced tomatoes, coconut milk, tomato paste, garam masala, cumin, coriander, turmeric, salt, and pepper in the slow cooker.

Stir to mix.

Cover and cook on low for 6-8 hours or on high for 3-4 hours until chicken is cooked through and flavours are thoroughly mixed.

Serve hot over cooked rice, topped with fresh cilantro.

C. Slow Cooker Vegetarian Chilli

A substantial and nutritious vegetarian chilli filled with beans, vegetables, and delicious spices, cooked to perfection in a slow cooker

Ingredients:

2 cans (15 oz each) kidney beans, drained and rinsed

1 can (15 oz) black beans, drained and rinsed

1 can (15 oz) corn kernels, drained

1 onion, chopped

1 red bell pepper, chopped

1 green bell pepper, chopped

3 cloves garlic, minced

1 can (28 oz) chopped tomatoes

2 cups vegetable broth

2 teaspoons chili powder

1 tablespoon cumin

1 teaspoon paprika

Salt and pepper to taste

Optional toppings: shredded cheese, sour cream, minced cilantro, sliced green onions

Instructions:

Place kidney beans, black beans, corn, onion, bell peppers, garlic, diced tomatoes, vegetable broth, chilli powder, cumin, paprika, salt, and pepper in the slow cooker.

Stir to mix.

Cover and simmer on low for 6-8 hours or on high for 3-4 hours until vegetables are soft and flavours are thoroughly integrated.

Serve hot, topped with your favourite toppings.

Chapter 18

Meal Planning Tips and Strategies for Long-Term Blood Sugar Management

Meal planning is a critical element of maintaining blood sugar levels for those with diabetes. By carefully selecting nutritious foods and regulating portion sizes, it's feasible to accomplish long-term blood sugar control and improve overall health.

II. Understanding Nutritional Needs

A. Overview of Macronutrients

To maintain stable blood sugar levels, it's vital to understand the significance of macronutrients in the diet. Carbohydrates, proteins, and lipids each play a unique function in regulating blood sugar:

Carbohydrates: These are the main source of energy for the body and have the most significant impact on blood sugar levels. Choose complex carbs with a low glycemic index to prevent blood sugar rises.

Proteins: Protein-rich diets assist enhance satiety and slow down the absorption of carbs. Include lean sources of protein such as poultry, fish, tofu, and lentils in your meals.

Fats: Healthy fats are crucial for overall health and can help balance blood sugar levels. Opt for sources of unsaturated fats like avocados, nuts, seeds, and olive oil.

B. Importance of Fiber and Micronutrients

In addition to macronutrients, it's essential to focus on fibre and micronutrients:

Fibre: High-fibre foods help slow down the absorption of carbohydrates and promote digestive health. Include plenty of fruits, veggies, whole grains, and legumes in your diet.

Micronutrients: Vitamins and minerals play a key part in overall health and well-being. Aim to consume a range of nutrient-dense foods to ensure you're reaching your micronutrient demands.

II. Practical Meal Planning Tips

A. Portion Control and Balanced Meals

Maintaining portion control and balancing meals is crucial to maintaining blood sugar levels:

Portion Sizes: Use visual clues, measurement equipment, or portion control plates to manage portion sizes efficiently.

Balanced Meals: Aim to incorporate a balance of carbohydrates, proteins, and fats in each meal to help stabilise blood sugar levels and induce satiety.

B. Meal Timing and Frequency

Eating regular meals and snacks throughout the day can help reduce blood sugar rises and crashes:

Meal Timing: Spread meals and snacks equally throughout the day to maintain stable blood sugar levels. Aim for consistent eating times to build a pattern.

Snacking: Choose healthy snacks that contain a combination of carbohydrates, proteins, and fats to help maintain blood sugar levels constant between meals.

C. Smart Carbohydrate Choices

Selecting carbs with a low glycemic index/load can help decrease blood sugar fluctuations:

Low-Glycemic Carbohydrates:
Choose whole grains, fruits, vegetables, and legumes that have a lesser impact on blood sugar levels.

Fiber-Rich Foods: Opt for fibre-rich foods like oatmeal, quinoa, berries, and beans to help slow down the absorption of carbohydrates.

III. Practical Meal Planning Strategies

A. Weekly Meal Prep and Batch Cooking

Meal prep and bulk cooking can save time and ensure you have healthful meals readily available:

Planning: Set some time each week to plan your meals and snacks. Make a grocery list and fill up on essentials.

Preparation: Prep ingredients in advance, such as washing and cutting vegetables or cooking grains and proteins. Store ready components in containers for simple assembly.

B. Recipe Modification and Substitution

Modify recipes to make them more diabetes-friendly by lowering sugar, fat, and refined carbohydrates:

Ingredient Swaps: Substitute ingredients with healthier alternatives, such as using whole grain flours, natural sweeteners, and lean meats.

Recipe Adjustments: Adjust recipes to lessen sugar and fat levels while still keeping flavour and texture.

Experiment with herbs, spices, and flavourings to increase taste.

C. Flexibility and Adaptability

Be flexible and adaptable with meal planning to accommodate shifting schedules and preferences:

Customization: Build a library of diverse recipes that can be adjusted to suit your tastes and dietary demands.

 range: Incorporate a range of meals into your meal plan to ensure you're achieving your nutritional needs and avoiding boredom.

IV. Incorporating Physical Activity

A. Importance of Physical Activity

Regular exercise is vital for regulating blood sugar levels and increasing overall health:

Benefits: Exercise helps improve insulin sensitivity, manage blood sugar levels, and lower cardiovascular risk.

Types of activity: Include aerobic activity, strength training, and flexibility exercises in your routine for a well-rounded fitness program.

B. Strategies for Incorporating Exercise

Find ways to incorporate physical activity into your everyday routine:

Scheduling: Schedule exercise sessions at times that work best for you, whether it's in the morning, afternoon, or evening.

Enjoyment: Choose activities that you enjoy and that meet your fitness level and interests. Whether it's walking, cycling, swimming, or dancing, choose things that make you feel good.

Meal planning is a valuable tool for managing blood sugar levels and increasing general health and well-being. By following these practical guidelines and methods, you can take control of your diet and lifestyle to achieve long-term blood sugar management and live your best life with diabetes.